How To

Lose Weight

In An

OverWeight

World

Peter LeGrove

This Is My Story About How I Went From Over A 41 Inch Waist To Under A 36 Inch Waist In Four Months

Disclaimer

Your Free Book

As a way of saying thank you for buying my book I'm offering you a free book.

This book "How To Add Qualifications To Your CV Using FREE Courses" is about what you can learn over the internet for free. It shows you where to go to get Certificates of Accomplishment that you can add to your CV.

Click here and you will be taken to another page where you can download the free book.

Get Your FREE book here

Who Will Benefit From This Book

If you are trying to lose weight or knock a few inches off your waistline, then this book could be what you are looking for. It goes into detail about how I tightened up my waist over a 4 month period. I went from over a 41 inch waist to under 36 and it was not easy. I did my own exercise schedule and made a few changes to my diet, amongst a few other things, that all helped to knock off the inches. The book goes into detail about the changes I made and the different exercises I tried. Also the book covers diet, sleeping and not overdoing the exercises. If you are thinking about getting into shape or trying too and getting very few results then this little book might show you where you are going wrong. There is a bit more to losing belly fat that sweating it out with a lot of huffing and puffing for about half an hour a day .

When I started out trying to get a better waistline, I thought doing an ab workout and a few other exercises everyday would make a difference. I will admit I did get fitter and over time I would have knocked off the extra inches but it didn't happen overnight.

This book is not about an exercise schedule you should follow to lose weight. It is about finding out about what you need to do, and changing things around to get better results. There is a lot of information on the internet and I just sorted out the little bits that helped me. But it all boils down to putting in the effort everyday or every other day and doing it. That means sweating it out in your bedroom or in the gym. It is up to you.

How To Use This Book

This book is about change and about wanting to change and actually doing something about it. It is also a do it yourself book. Whether you clear some space in your bedroom, or the lounge or go to the gym it is up to you. You do not have a personal trainer showing you what to do and keeping tabs on you. You are your own personal trainer, and therefore you have to push yourself. You have to make time and you have to do it. You should allow half an hour to an hour a day when you start out, just to get into the swing of things. Most of that time will be spent recovering from the few exercises you are trying to do. And then over a short time it will be the other way round. Where you do more exercises than recovery.

Don't push yourself too far too fast. First you have to increase your fitness levels to a point where you can do the exercises, then you will start to see and feel a difference. So first up you'll be huffing and puffing and sweating away for a very short time as you realize how unfit you really are. It is only after you get fitter, then the benefits click in and you start to feel fitter. But it takes a lot of sweat to get to this point. And you have to keep pushing yourself and pushing yourself a littler further each week. But don't overdo it as you will be the person with the sore muscles.

To start buy a mat to do your exercises on, then check out the links to the workout videos. Pick an easy one to start and away you go. If you are still feeling good try another. Do two different sessions back to back, one standing exercises and the other on the mat. If the exercises are too mean give them a miss until you get fitter, then try them out. Just get started that is the main thing.

What Is In This Book

Why You Should Get Fit

Exercise And Inflammation

Where I Was

My First Attempt

The New Routine With The Videos

Now Onto Goals And Goal Setting

Documentary "Fat Verses Sugar"

Changing My Food Intake And Schedule

Lack Of Sleep Can Cause Weight Gain

Doing Exercises In Other Cities

Summary Time

Things You Can Do

Articles From The Internet Mentioned In The Book

Why You Should Get Fit

There are many benefits to getting and keeping fit as you age. Lately there has been a lot of published research on how exercise throughout your life can keep your brain and body in better health. Or you can take pills and put up with the side effects

One of the best ways to get into the swing of fitness, is just to start reading about it on the internet or gets some books from the library. And read regularly so you implant the new ideas in your mind. The more you read about it the more you think you can do it. Also now with the modern generation watch the videos on the internet. Here you have to be careful that you are watching something that will be helpful. Get your kids to look up a few good videos, especially if they are into fitness. My daughter set me up with a number of good videos to watch. My daughter used to do her workout watching a video. That is the modern generation so why not join it. This is the start. Just doing this, reading regularly keeps the idea of fitness right in front of you and it will not take to long to switch over from the thinking to the doing. You will start to think 'maybe I can' as opposed to 'I cant' without even trying.

Now when you do start, do not go overboard and do some some damage. Just take it slow. The best way to start is just doing exercises at home. Do easy exercises first like 'the plank.' Here your forearm from your elbows to your hands are on the ground as well as your toes and your back is straight, from your shoulders to your toes. That is the plank position but to start rest on your knees not your toes until you get a bit more strength. All you have to do is stay in that position for as long as you can, no movement required, until you collapse in a heap on the floor. Before you collapse turn your face sideways so if you do hit the floor you do not damage your nose or teeth. Better still put a pillow on the floor where your face will land just in case you collapse. It is best to get a soft yoga mat to do your exercises on, except in summer the mat can get covered in sweat then it can be get quite slippery. 'The plank' is a good exercise at least it gets you on the floor and you don't have to do anything, except look at the clock and see how long you can stay in the plank position. It is not easy to stay in the plank position for a long period of time so don't overdo it. Your stomach muscles will give way first. Then after you are comfortable with the plank you can start moving into the 'push up' position, count to 10 then go back to the plank position, count to 10, then back up to the push up position. All you are doing is going from your forearms touching the ground to your hands on the ground and your arms are straight up and down to your shoulders. No push ups just yet, you need a bit more strength in your arms before you start those. While on the mat we'll try an easy exercise on your back. On your back with your hands either under your head or on the floor beside you, and the soles of your feet flat on the ground with your knees up in the air. All you are doing is moving your knees to your chest and back down again, these are 'reverse crunches' and they are a lot easier than lifting your upper body up to your knees. Do as many as you can but don't overdo it, you don't want to be all sore the next day because if that happens it will be more difficult to get you started again. You do not want to be a speed racer, just do things slowly and you will do less damage to your body. Every time you do exercises you actually do damage your body, so always give your body time to recover. The people who have problems do not give their body time to recover, or they go like a bat out of hell and all they are doing is increasing inflammation in their body and that is not good. So don't be silly just gradually build up what you can do. If you have sore muscles or are sore anywhere don't do any exercise, just wait till your body recovers. If you want to do exercise everyday do different exercises. One day on the mat and the next day on your feet and possible go for a job the day after that. There are a lot of good standing exercises to do but I like squats. They are easy, just stand there with your back straight, then start bending your knees and lower your body as far as you can and stand up again. Now do as many as you can. Squats are usually on the list of exercises you need to do. With all exercise to build muscle you must go slow and steady, you only build muscle when your muscles start pinging or when you start straining. You don't build as much muscle when you go fast and you are increasing lactic acid in your body which is not good. So do everything slowly and steadily.

Now to get started you have to make the time and it is easier in summer when you can go for a run or do exercises outside. Or get a cheap gym membership and go for it. You should get into a routine and this way you know when you will do your exercises. Just start with squats and other easy to do exercises like lunges. Just standing exercises first. Then get a yoga mat and start on the floor. Even if you can't do too many the first few times you will slowly build up. Like when you start doing push ups start on your knees first until you are comfortable then move to your toes. When you start don't try to do too much, just get into the swing of things and as you get better add to the exercises. When you start exercising after any exercise sessions you will have sore spots around your body. The best way is to not go overboard or you could cause too much inflammation in your body and that is not a good thing. So do a different exercise regime that uses different muscles. Like one day do exercises standing up and the next day on the mat. When you have pain stop. A lot of times you will not feel the pain until afterwards but when you are running you will feel it immediately. If you pull a muscle or have any pain stop because if you don't your recovery time could be longer and you need your legs. The worst injury I had was when I damaged my Plantar fasciitis. That is the bottom of your foot or the sole of your feet. That is very painful and the only way to stop the pain is to walk and stretch your heel. Just getting out of bed was a mission but after walking round for a bit it gets better. I've damaged both soles of my feet at different time and I know I did one while running. I was trying out High Intensity Interval Training by sprinting and jogging and I don't know what I did but it hurt like hell and I had to stop running and limp home. After a few days I could still do skipping no problem because when you are skipping you are stretching the sole of you feet and that is what you need to do to make it better. Also another problem that crops up is cramps so I take a magnesium supplement and that helps. Sometimes my legs cramp up really bad especially at night and that is not good. So when you start exercising take it easy don't overdo it because that is when you have problems. It might be an idea to tell your doctor that you are going to start exercising so he can keep an eye on you so you don't cause any problems. But you have to find time and then get into it.

Exercise And Inflammation

When you start exercising you have to know something about inflammation as it will affect you and sometimes in not very good ways. Here I will go through how inflammation has affected me while I was exercising. Inflammation can affect you in some weird and wonderful ways and some of the time you just don't know why. For example I had a pain in my knee for about 4 days,. I don't remember damaging my knee or spraining it or anything it just started hurting and it didn't stop. It was just a low level pain in the background so I could still get around alright. These things happen with exercise and inflammation. Also it could have been my body's way of telling me to slow down so listen to your body.

My foot has been hurting for months now so I am used to that, but this time my knee started hurting, and that is a new one. Even if I just rested my arm on my knee it would start to hurt. I was starting to wonder what it was, I thought it might be arthritis or something like that then it vanished. Also it might have been because I was limping a little so I might have put more strain on my knee and that caused the problem, but we will never know as it went away.

Now the worst minor injury you can get from exercise is damaging your planter fascitis in your foot. I damaged mine sprinting across the football field. Your planter fascitis is the tendon that runs from the back of your heel under your foot to your toes, and you don't want to damage it as it hurts like hell and it is very difficult to get comfortable with this aliment. Mainly because you are on your feet most of the time and when you drive it can make it worse. And that is something you also don't want because when it is resting it hurts the most. In the mornings after sleeping you can hardly put your foot on the floor it hurts so much. You have to stretch it and walk on it to make it feel better. And hopefully after a couple of months it will be back to normal. Your planter fascitis is very easy to damage as I said I did mine while sprinting and if you read the literature that is the most common way to damage it. A damaged planter fascitis will slow you down. Now because of my planter fascitis I couldn't run or do too many exercises so I don't know if that was a bad thing or not.

Another time when inflammation took over was when I somehow hurt my foot and didn't know it. My planter fascitis was nearly back to normal but my foot just swelled up big time like a balloon. I could hardly put it on the floor and my toes were stuck out like fingers when you blow up a plastic glove. I didn't know what to do I couldn't walk to the car let alone drive to the hospital. So I propped my foot up on pillows so it was elevated and just waited. It didn't hurt at all but it looked terrible. Whenever I have problems with inflammation I take Vitamin C in large doses, like 1000mgs every two hours, and that seems to keep me alive. But is only when I have swelling or inflammation pain, not all the time. Also I mix Tumeric with my breakfast drink as that helps to lower inflammation levels or so the natural health people say. Anyway the next morning it had started to go down and by lunchtime I could walk again with a limp, To this day I still don't know what caused my foot to swell up. That is what inflammation can do to you, so expect it.

Where I Was

Starting waist measurement - 41 and a half inches around my waist

I've been a pretty slim line sort of dude for a long time. The first time I had a problem with the flab I also had a problem with the beer. I mean I was very pear shaped then. I was also a driver and that is not the most energetic job on the planet. So I packed on the beef sitting on my butt all day. Anyway I got that under control and was back to a slim line dude once again. This time I was doing a job on my feet all day, so I didn't have to worry too much about packing on the pounds. And the job was such a job that I sometimes forgot to eat, and it was nothing for me to go all day without eating anything, just drinking green tea. Anyway I got into this intermittent fasting craze that seemed to be taking hold of the healthy world. I didn't really plan it that way. I just fell into that pattern and some days I would go without eating all day until about 9 oclock at night. And it didn't worry me at all. I wasn't even trying intermittent fasting I just ended up doing it. I would try and go two days a week without food, and had no problems at all with food or lack off. On top of all this I'd ride my bike around most days, and do two nights a week doing self defense and fitness. I got into this high intensity fitness style of exercise, where I was peddling my bike as hard as I could for about 30 seconds then coasting for 30 seconds. This way I wouldn't wear myself out so fast and I felt good after doing this type of exercise. Instead of peddling like mad until I collapsed.

This was my life for about three years. Then it all changed. I lost my job. The company shut down and I started looking for another job. This time I got a job sitting on my butt all day in front of a computer. And to top it off I had to move to a new city. And it was winter do I stopped riding my bike. As I was in a new city I never quite got back into riding the bike so much. I tried it out a few times but couldn't get into the rhythm. Losing a job has a psychological impact on a few people and I was one of them. In the old town I had a lot of friends and I had a good life with all the groups I belonged too. In the new town I knew nobody and it was pretty hard to fit in. So I resorted to eating more junk food and processed food. And because my salary was not as good as before, I was eating cheaper quality food. And if I saw something on special I would buy a lot of it. And that is how I ended up buying three packets of meat pies with a devious use-by-date. These were three packets of six pies each, so I ended up with 18 pies and no room in the freezer. So it was two pies a day until I finished them. That is when I noticed I was starting to pack on the pounds. I was getting a beer gut without the beer. This was only eight months into my new lifestyle of sitting on my butt all day eating anti depression food that tasted really good. I love pies, and if they go on special again I'll buy another packet but this time not three packets. The reason I brought three packets was because the brand was good, and I hadn't eaten pies for a long time. They were not something that went on special very often, so I made the most of it. I had stopped my intermittent fasted, riding my bike and eating reasonable healthy food. So I was starting to reap the benefits of a very unhealthy lifestyle and that was showing on my waistline.

Another change that happened with the new job and the new town was it was afternoon work. So I'd end up going to bed at 2 to 3 in the morning. Before when I used to do the afternoon shift it was the healthiest time of my life. I used to go to bed after midnight and sleep as long as I liked with no alarm to wake me up. Now that doesn't happen. I'm a morning person and this threw my whole life into turmoil. I went from getting a good night's sleep to getting next to none. I even tried split sleeping to try and catch some sleep in the afternoon. Didn't work. I got a black face mask to keep out the light, but that was only touch and go. It kept the light out and I did manage to sleep longer, but it was not every night.

I raided the health food shop, and came away with an armload of sleeping supplements. I'm still working on some of them. Some are certified useless and others, well the jury is still out on those. Some do actually work but I can't rely on them. That means they don't work every time, just sometimes and I haven't worked out why. For me to start taking pill things was not good. Then along came daylight saving and that completely throw my circadian rhythm out of whack. What little sleep I was getting before just got less, and I was at my wits end. I have had problems with sleeping before, but this was the worst I could remember. Before I could live with it and it didn't worry me so much, but now things were different. I read somewhere on the internet, that sleep and weight gain as well as night shift are somehow all related.

My life was a complete mess. I went from a healthy, relaxed lifestyle to what I am in now, in less than a year, like 8 months and it was getting worse. It was so bad or I thought it was, that I started praying, something I hadn't done for years. Things were not good in my life. I was praying for a good night's sleep and the jury is still out on that one too. In the Bible it says something like "Pray as though you have received and you will receive." So I used to pray "Thank you God for 8 hours sleep last night" even though I only got 3 to 5 hours. I would say that when I woke up over and over again before I looked at the time. Sometimes I would actually fall back to sleep again and wake up after 8 o clock which was very unusual, so maybe it did work, but so far I'm still waiting for 8 hours uninterrupted sleep. Gotta try everything, it all helps. Can't rely on pills all the time.

My First Attempt

Anyway back to trying to get rid of the pot gut. After checking my profile in the full length mirror it was time to do something. So I started on a very small exercise program, as many press ups as I could do and that was not very many, as well as sit ups, leg raises and squats. These were some of the same exercises I used to do at the self defense class I used to go to in the old city. After two weeks of doing these there was no difference, so I added in running around the football field two times, twice or three times a week. Things were not good. Also somewhere on the internet it said that internal parasites could cause weight gain even though I was under the impression it was the other way round. So I popped an anti worm pill, as I have had problems with internal parasites before. Also I started eating raw pumpkin seeds as they help rid your body of parasites. And I added a few cloves of raw Garlic to the mix as that is supposed to do something about parasites. Garlic is one of the few things that can keep you awake, so I had to balance between going out and not eating garlic before trying to get some sleep. You cannot eat garlic before you go to work because you will stink out the whole office. Not really good for promotions.

Also there was something about your thyroid and sleep. I'm not sure of the connection but thyroid function and sleep go together. So it was time to start painting myself with iodine to keep my thyroid function up to par. I went to my GP doctor and he gave me some Melathonin which was supposed to help me to stay asleep. The jury is still out on that one too. Next stop was with my natural health medicine man. He said my magnesium levels were probably out of sync as I was probably taking too much magnesium, so he put me on a mixture of magnesium and potassium. And hopefully this would balance out the magnesium levels in my body. It didn't change my sleeping patterns at all.

Even though I had started out on a quest to drop a few pounds, the sleep thing was worrying me more than the extra pounds. So somehow the quest to drop the pounds morphed into a quest to get a good night's sleep. And they were both somehow related.

Next up I had to look at my diet and eating habits. I had completely given up on the intermittent fasting but I still managed to eat twice a day. But this time round I was eating a lot of biscuits, lots of cheese, lots of dates, and my eating times were very irregular. Also before I lived in the countryside and I used to drink a lot of farm milk that is milk straight from the cow. And now I couldn't get that. I was still drinking lots of green and black tea. Probably more black tea than before. On three or four days a week I would drink about two liters of tea so I was very hydrated, the same as before. I have a problem with gluten, it seems to be heredity as my bother and sister both have problems with gluten. My brother has serious problems with it and my sister not so much. With me it is quite handy to have, as gluten puts me to sleep. And I knew if I could find some really good heavy duty gluten bread I could pick up a couple of extra hour's sleep in the afternoon, as it would only put me to sleep for a couple of hours max. For some reason, possible related to my sugar levels balancing out, I would end up wide awake after a couple of hours. Because of this gluten problem I don't eat bread very much. If good quality bread is on special at the supermarket I will buy it, but usually the only bread I buy is the cheapest to feed the birds.

Now to somehow get my life back to some sort of reasonable living pattern, I brought a skipping rope and an exercise mat. I figured I could get back into high intensity exercises using a skipping rope and fast slow running, instead of just running around the football field. My daughter showed me a few youtube videos about exercises for abs, so I would have a program to follow. And I was good to go. The first attempt at watching the videos and doing them didn't amount to much so I'll have to rearrange things. It takes a while to get into a new pattern. What to keep and what to change. I'm still doing my mini morning routine with the skipping, but I'll start to bring in the new exercises from the video. My main problem, is I trashed my back in a car smash many years ago and I still have issues with some exercises. So I do them as best I can. At the moment I am 41 and a half inches around my waist. A far cry from the somewhere between 34 and 36 that I usually am. I am 71 inches (5 foot 11 inches) tall so my height to circumference is a bit out of whack. My first goal is to get back to a 34 to 36 inch waist. This way I should end up with some abs. At the moment it is just beer gut without the beer.

The New Routine With The Videos

According to the Doctor Mercola website my ideal waist to my height should be 32 and a half inches. I have never been that slim for years. At the moment I am at the top end of the overweight scale or at the bottom end of the obese scale. Not a good place to be. I filled in Dr Mercola's Nutritional Typing questionnaire and I am a Mixed Type. So I follow his suggestions on what to eat. Another website on exercise and health that I like to follow is Craig Ballantyne from Early To Rise. This is one of his products here http://6minutestoskinny.com. If I can't figure out my weight pretty soon I'll see what he can do.

The first morning I had lined up three 10 minute videos and started out on the floor doing reverse crunches and trying to touch my toes with my legs stuck up in the air. That was quite difficult for me as my back was still pretty stiff after being in plaster for around 6 months. And as it was a back injury I had lowered mobility, making some of the exercises quite difficult. But I persevered and sweated and puffed my way through the first 10 minutes. Then I moved onto the second video which was a series of 45 second exercises for another 10 minutes. I spent most of the time on the mat breathing heavy and not doing to much. The last video was standing exercises and they were pretty easy to do. After half an hour of bumbling through the exercises I had hardly built up a sweat but I was pretty puffed, Some of the exercises I couldn't finish as my body was using new muscles and I usually didn't exercise for half an hour.

The second attempt was a bit more organized but only lasted 20 minutes. I didn't do any standing ab exercises. I started off with push ups and straight crunches, as I wanted to get them out of the road first. Then I went onto reverse crunches and body raises. Here I stick my legs up in the air and try and touch my toes, easier said that done.

Now it was onto leg scissors and back to reverse crunches and body raises. Next up it was ab side raises where I put my right arm past my left knee and then my left arm past my left knee. Now onto knee raises, alternating legs. Then the alarm on the washing machine went off meaning 20 minutes was up. This time I took a rest when I changed exercises but I didn't break out into sweat or puffed too much, just a bit of heavy breathing. And to finish off I did squats. Here I did as many exercises as I could and to be honest I couldn't do too many. After I finished hanging out the washing I did a little bit of semi intensive running. I would run for about 40 seconds then rest for another 20 to 30 seconds and do another round. I did 4 rounds. Got the heart pumping a bit faster but I don't think it got over 100 beats a minute. I like doing the high intensity exercises on the stationary bike, as that has a heart monitor and a timer. Here I have no stationary bike, just a skipping rope and a pair of running shoes, so the rest is guess work.

After a week I am slowly getting into the swing of things. This time I added in side raises, then I run for around the football field a few times. Tomorrow I'll time myself and see how long I actually run. The running bit is the only part I'm getting better at and now I can run a little longer.

Now I have been pretty consistent lately. My exercise routine takes about 20 minutes, including breathing stops. I'm amazed at how unfit I am. I still have to stop for a rest and a breather quite regularly. Some of the exercises I have boosted up to do more but most I'm still struggling. Also I try to run for as long as I can and skip for about 5 minutes. I do the exercises everyday if possible but I only run and skip when it is not raining.

But after doing all this nothing has happened I'm still the same size. I still can't do many exercises and I do lots of heavy breathing and lying on the mat recovering.

So now I have to look at my diet. I've started doing a bit of fasting lately, but nothing like before. I belong to the school that believes, you burn fat by not eating for long periods of time. But I do have a fetish for biscuits. I only buy biscuits on special but there are always some on special. Usually I try to go as long as possible without eating solid food in the mornings. Because my schedule is all screwed up I go to bed about two in the morning. Then after I get up I try to go all day without food. I just drink heaps of green and black tea. On some days I would drink around 2 liters easily. That is usually my day.

Now Onto Goals And Goal Setting

I see goals in the lose weight get fit sites like "I will lose 10 lbs in 3 months and look trim etc etc". When you get stuck into dropping pounds and getting fit, you suddenly realize it is not easy. And if you don't make your goal you could get disheartened and give up. Very easy to do. To survive dropping pounds you have to basically change your life style, and keep the changes. If you expect the end result without doing anything then you are just hoping.

My goals are really simple. "I do my morning exercises a minimum of four times each week" This way it is up to me I can control that but I can't control the fat loss. So it puts the ball in your court so as to speak. With this goal my first exercise regime didn't seem to do anything so I changed it. But the goal stayed the same.

Also after I started running I started off saying "I would run around the football field once" and then when I got better at running and more fitter I went up to twice. I just added onto the existing goal. I was not chasing a goal that could very well be out of my control. Maybe I'm a control freak. The same with press ups. I started off at about five, and added to it. Now I am up to fifteen and some days I can't even do that. Going from 5 push ups to 10 push ups is not very difficult, but going from 10 to 15 is and it takes a long time. Don't expect miracles jut keep plodding on.

The other goals are to do with eating. I used to fast two days a week. Because of my life style it was easy to do. But now things have changed and it is difficult to try and fast, but I am working on it. Also eating fast food and eating out are controllable goals. Or even what you eat. You could set a goal like "I will eat three salads a week, every week." Controlling the outcome can be difficult but keeping the input under control is something you can do. One thing some goal experts recommend, is you find an accountability person and you tell this person or persons your goals, and they will help you keep them. I don't like that idea so no one knows my goals. I do hand write them down everyday in a notebook, so I can keep track of what I am doing. I do not copy the goals from the day before, I always write them down afresh in case they have changed from the day before. Goals do change and this way you can keep track of what you are achieving, and what is not working.

To keep on track you need to update your time management skills, as you are adding to your time. If you have a lot of spare time it is no problem, but if you are stretched then you have to book in your new schedule. Actually I had very little problem fitting it all in. I'm free nearly all day so it is no problem to fit in my morning exercise routine, and I could run around the football park any time I like. All up I had to find an hour extra a day but I could split up the hour. For skipping I just fitted that in any time. At the start my day routine was pretty jumbled but it evolved over time, and things got changed around pretty regularly. Now for me it was easy to get into the swing of things, but you might have to change a few things around. Also with push ups you can do them any time, before lunch after lunch, whenever. They are easy to do anywhere and you can do as many or as few as you can. If you can do push ups 3 or 4 times a day you will make more progress. I tried to do 10 push ups each time but sometimes I couldn't even do that.

Now if you have a major goal, one that is the main reason for doing exercises and going on a diet then you will have less problems finding time and changing your habits. That is the driving force behind you that will keep you going. If you do not have a serious enough goal then it could be a struggle. Usually it is your doctor saying if you do not get into shape you will have problems in the future. Or you wake up one day alone and you decide it is time to find somebody else. That is a very strong motivator, and you have to get into shape to make yourself appealing to the opposite sex. And you never know you might find someone in the gym. Which would be a plus as you could train together.

I was tired of being by myself so it was time to get back into shape and start hitting the dating sites to try and find somebody to be with. And getting back into shape is not the easiest thing to do so I had to persevere. And also I needed to get into shape because as you get older the fitter you are the healthier you are or so the natural health people say. And there is some truth in exercise is the best medicine so I'll see what happens. I'm quite lucky now I have no serious health issues and I'm not on any prescription meds at the moment.

The reason why you want to get into shape and drop a few pounds is the driving force behind you driving yourself on, until you get addicted to the exercises and the pain and the sweat. At that point you will have trouble slowing down and stopping. But to get to this point you will need to be working out about 5 times a week. You will need to be doing some pretty serious, heavy duty pushing yourself to the limit exercises to get to that point. And then you will see the changes. And you need a routine time schedule to follow, so time management is the key.

At the moment I'm not at that point yet. I am increasing the number of times I do most exercises and I still rest before changing to another exercise. I'm still doing about 20 minutes of exercises and a bit of running and some skipping during the day. And I still have to force myself to get started. But that will change as I get better at it. I had a wake up call last weekend when I was staying at my brother's house. All his kids are very into fitness, like they go to the gym at 6 o clock every morning. And this time they were all going for an uphill run, and if I was a bit fitter I would have gone with them. I had to turn it down as I was not in their league, but next time I should be.

Anyway now for an update on the sleeping pills. The ones I brought at the supermarket seem to be the best. I can usually get six hours sleep out of them. The Melatonin only give me about five and a half hours, while if I take nothing I'll be lucky if I get four hours. And for some unknown reason I can't seem to have a nap in the afternoon, like I did before. I have a lie down but I don't sleep. Things are still not good on the sleeping front. I can't say I'm working on it, as I am slowly running out of options. I don't know if lack of sleep is holding me back, but I am still the same weight and the tape measure hasn't moved. And I'm doing exercises nearly everyday and running and skipping.

Documentary "Fat Verses Sugar"

I read somewhere on the internet after doing a health quiz that I was not eating enough. I completely wrote it off as rubbish as I can go all day without eating. But there might be something in that as I am not losing any weight. I was under the impression, that to burn fat you should try not to eat solid food as long as possible after getting up after sleeping. And since my eating habits are totally screwed up because of my lifestyle change, I don't seem to have a pattern of when to eat during the day. I don't know when I eat. I usually don't eat when I m hungry, I usually eat when I think about it. Or more likely when something in the fridge is ready to go off, or is getting pretty close to its use-by-date. I don't like waste. Anyway I don't think I'll change my eating habits at the moment.

I watched the documentary "Fat Verses Sugar" .Fat verses Sugar about 2 twin brothers who wanted to find out what was worse, sugar or fat, so one twin only ate sugar food while the other only ate fat food. Actually the one who only ate sugar had better insulin control but he only lost one kilo of body mass, half from muscle mass and half from fat. While the twin on fat lost around 3.5kgs of body mass, 2 kgs of muscle mass and 1.5 kgs of fat, but had problems with his insulin levels and was heading into prediabetic territory. Sounds really strange, the twin on sugar had better control of insulin, and the twin on fat was heading into dangerous territory with insulin. When on a high sugar diet your body manages to control insulin better. But when on a fat diet your body has to produce more insulin and that could lead to problems. And that was only after a month on the fat diet. The doctor did say while on a long term sugar diet that could cause problems in the future, but he recommended to stop the fat diet immediately. I have serious problems believing that as I eat more fat than sugar, and I was under the impression sugar was the problem. But what is causing my weight gain is most likely eating too many biscuits, as the program came to the conclusion that a combination of around 50% fat and 50% sugar in food was a mixture we were biologically not evolved to eat. Therefore our brains could not send any signals to stop us eating this food so we don't know when to stop. And that about sums up my biscuit eating habits, I open a packet and I finish it in one sitting. I just can't seem to stop myself. Not the healthiest way to eat but they taste good,

Now what I have to do now is find out how to lose body fat without losing muscle mass. After checking out the literature online, it suddenly dawned on me that my eating habits were what was causing me not to lose any weight. Intermittent fasting was my big problem. When I was working on my feet intermittent fasting twice a week helped keep me trim. But now I wanted to lose belly fat and not what limited muscle I had and fasting was having the opposite effect. I wasn't losing too much belly fat as I was not eating enough. I needed more protein in my diet, and it seemed I needed carbohydrate after exercising.

I eat lots of fat, like I cook in coconut oil and I eat a tablespoon a day of coconut oil. I also use lard and butter for cooking. I will not eat margarine or cook in vegetable oil except for olive oil. There is some debate over what is a healthy fat and what isn't. The fats I like to use are the ones that have not been over processed. Most vegetable oils do not come under this category so I don't use them too much. Also there is no sugar or artificial sweeteners in my house only honey. I asked the lawnmower man in for a cup of tea after mowing the lawns and he asked for sugar. I realized then we had no sugar in the house so I put honey in his tea. I don't eat very much processed food at all except for some tinned foods like baked beans, beetroot and tomatoes. In winter I kinder get stuck into tinned foods as there are not too many vegetables around. Not a very healthy substitute especially when you add in the biscuits.

After watching the documentary I was surprised to find the fat diet was not the healthiest. When he lost the weight, he lost under 2 kgs of fat and the rest was muscle. So he lost 2 kgs of muscle therefore he lost muscle mass. Maybe that is my problem. I don't want to lose muscle just belly fat, but I still can't seem to lose weight even though I exercise regularly. Maybe I should boost up the running. Lately it has been raining so I haven't been out for a run. As soon as it dries out a bit I start running again.

Well when it stopped raining I kinder went overboard, doing some serious running and then I started doing high intensity skipping. I was skipping hard for 30 seconds then I jogged for another 30 seconds and started all over again. I have been skipping for a long time but never really hard. But this time I hurt my back. I don't know how it happened, but it is quite painful and I have to modify my morning routine. I can't do toe touches anymore but the other exercises I can still do. Maybe the toe touches put my back out. Now I am doing more exercises on my feet not on my back. Like a set of lunges that I will modify into a kicking lunge. I'll bring in some side lunges and deep pile squats.

Changing My Food Intake And Schedule

I checked out the internet on this burn fat not muscle, and to summarize it all I would say I need to eat more protein after exercising. But this Doctor says we eat too much protein and we should eat less protein. He recommends around 40 to 70 grams of protein a day for the average person, which is lower than what the fitness people recommend. As I eat a lot of meat I would say my protein levels should be too high. Usually I eat nothing in the morning and sometimes I only eat once a day, and I thought that is a recipe for muscle burn, but it doesn't seem to be. After working out your body needs more energy, so if it runs out of easy fat to burn you end up burning muscle.

And I think that is what I am doing because I ended up with a sore back.

Also you need to lower your calorie intake. People in the know call this 'caloric deficit' meaning you have to eat less. This way you burn fat instead of burning food. I don't have to worry about my calorie intake as I don't over eat, even though I still go on biscuit binges occasionally. I have absolutely no idea how many calories I consume everyday. And I don't worry about it as I probably need to eat more. I found that after I started exercising I tended to eat less. I am also reasonable healthy. I don't eat too much processed food, I'm not into bread as I have a slight problem with gluten. And I probably eat too much fat meat. As far as I can work out my main problem is probably lack of food. And as I am doing more physical stuff I need the fat to stop burning muscle.

Anyway I did a serious change. I changed my exercise time to the afternoon. This way I can still not eat in the mornings and I should have enough protein in my body. So when I start exercising I shouldn't have to worry too much about muscle burn. Now I either run first or do my exercises first depending on how I feel. Also now I alternate which exercises I do each day. I always do push-ups, sit-ups, reverse crunches and toe touches and the rest change each day. I just try to keep it up for 20 minutes each time. If I run first, by the time I have walked home from the football field about 10 minutes, I have cooled off enough and my breathing is back to normal so I can go straight into exercises. The other way round if I do my exercises first, the 10 minute walk to the field is enough time to get my mind into running mode. I think this little change is more suited to my lifestyle. Now I don't need to change my eating habits to suit my exercise schedule. I'm just fitting everything in around my old lifestyle schedule.

Well it has finally happened I measured myself today and I am under 41 inches, so I have lost nearly an inch. Not bad for a month. It takes a while to get into the exercise thing, and now I have sorted out a schedule that doesn't impact my strange eating habits it is starting to have an effect. I just have to keep it up. Doing everything in the afternoon seems to be better as I do all the exercises in one hit. This way I can work up a sweat and actually feel like I am doing something.

I haven't checked my weight as I want to lose belly fat, and I am more interested in dropping the flab around my middle than how much I weigh. So I just keep the tape measure handy. The main reason I'm starting to slim down is I think, just doing the exercises. I've stopped worrying about losing muscle instead of fat. And I haven't changed my diet. One of the articles I read basically said we all eat too much protein, which is very possible as I eat meat everyday. One thing I have started, is to eat more eggs but that is mainly because I have a supply of free range eggs. And eggs are protein rich. Other than that the only change is the exercises, running and skipping. As I have got better at doing the exercises I can do more of them and I can exercise longer and run longer. And I think that is the key to losing the fat. The internet is a double edged sword with information overload. First I got the videos of the exercise to watch. Then I got a bit more into it by checking out the fat to muscle ratio, which I didn't really need too know. Now I just do the exercises and that is it.

I changed my exercise schedule a little bit as the weather started to warm up and it stopped raining. Now I run for about 20 minutes a day and do standing exercises only, like squats, lunges and burpees and finishing off with pushups and sit ups if I can still do them. Plus I'd try and do three kartas from my karate class. These are a standard routine, block / hit demonstration. And as I was doing them by myself, I could put as much energy and effort into them as I want. I didn't have to worry about hitting anybody, so I was hitting as hard as I could. And that takes a lot of effort. I was blending karate into some of the other exercises, like kick squats and punch squats. I tried doing kick lunges but I couldn't get into rhythm.

Now after doing all the exercises and running for 20 minutes around 5 times a week I would have thought it would start to have an effect. But so far l've only lost less than an inch around my waist. So I dived back into the internet to find some answers. And the sleep connection could be part of the problem. <u>Well according to this it does anyway.</u> But then again I have always had a problem with sleep, and only lately l've got a problem with the belly fat. But after digging a bit deeper I came up against testosterone. Now this might be a bigger part of the problem, as I have quite a few symptoms of lowered testosterone. But there is a silver lining here as one of the ways to increase testosterone levels is high intensity interval exercises. So now it is time to get back into high intensity interval exercises. I always liked doing them.

My high intensive interval training to date consisted off sitting on an exercise bike and peddling like mad for 30 seconds, then 30 seconds slow peddling. This way I could keep an eye on my pulse rate. I could get my pulse rate up to around 120 max. I just couldn't seem to get it higher. I could last about 10 minutes before I couldn't peddle anymore. When I first started I would run out of breath before my legs packed it in. But after I got my breath under control, I could peddle until my legs caved in.

With the running bit I used to run once around the football field, and with adding a new round every now and then I got up to 10 rounds in just over 20 minutes. Which I thought was pretty good. Now I wanted to do HIIT with the running. I could run one length on the football field in about 25 seconds. Then I would slow jog the short side of the field for about 30 seconds then I would run like mad again to the other side. Believe it or not I could only do 2 fast runs until I couldn't make it to the other side. And that was mainly because of breath not legs. I had to do something to control my breathing, it was my limiting factor. I would start off with a slow warm up jog around the field and I would end with another round.

Now I started looking at this Tabata HIIT out of Japan. This is pretty mean with 20 seconds hard slog and only 10 seconds recover, and then you are back into it again. The only trouble with this exercise is you have to be very fit to actually finish a four minute round. Even though I had been exercising for about 2 months I still was not fit, so I had serious problems just finishing a round. But it was something new to try and I knew one way to get fit was to keep doing exercises. Even with all the exercises I'm doing I'm still only lost a little over an inch. I am now under 40 inches, and it has taken a lot of effort to get there. I'm still not very fit even though I exercise quite regularly. I do self defense twice a week, and that is usually over an hour of hard slog. And the other days I do exercises around the house or on the mat. And now I have added sprinting as interval training, but I can't do very many of those until I nearly collapse.

Lack Of Sleep Can Cause Weight Gain

I still think my sleeping habits must play a large part in why I'm having trouble losing weight. And my sleeping habits have got worse lately. I used to get 6 hours a night but now for some unknown reason I can only manage 5 hours and I don't know why. That just started lately. Maybe there is more to losing weight than just doing exercises. I've managed to incorporate intermittent fasting into the mix and now I try to go 16 hours without food up to three times a week. At least some days I should be able to do over 20 hours without food, I might even make it to 24 hours without food at least twice a week. Anyway that is what is recommended. If anything I'm more healthy even though my goal of getting back to 34 to

36 around my waist is more difficult than I first imagined. Some people are extremely good at losing weight but not all. My friend at the gym pulled a muscle in his leg and was laid up for 6 weeks. He had packed on the pounds, but as soon as he got the all clear from his trainer he went on a 16 kilometer run. After 3 days of this he was back to his normal weight. For some people it is so easy.

I read this really depressing article about sleep and weight gain. Now I have always had trouble sleeping, and lately it has got worse. I now sleep around 5 hours before I wake up. And if I am lucky I also get a nap in the afternoon. Now I don't know why I've suddenly stopped sleeping. I eat a bit more healthier, that means less junk food and less food. In a nut shell when you have less sleep it affects two hormones. You end up with reduced leptin and elevated ghrelin. These differences in leptin and ghrelin are likely to increase appetite, possibly explaining why it is very difficult to lose weight when you have sleep problems. Leptin deficiency increases appetite and produces obesity while ghrelin is an appetite stimulator. So you can see, if you have increased ghrelin levels your appetite stimulator is working overtime so you will eat more. And that is all caused by lack of sleep. Now for the cruncher, sleep duration below 7.7 hours was associated with increased weight. I have never slept for over 7.7 hours for a long time, and I mean decades. And I'm not the only one. My friend is on call at his job and he can work anytime. When they call him he goes and he takes everything he can get, as he never knows when the next shift will be. And he has serious problems with weight and diabetes. And as he is not the most energetic person on the planet. His diabetes is getting out of control, even though his diet is very healthy. There is a lot more to losing weight than doing exercises and watching what you eat.

Things are looking good I had to do my belt up another notch so I knew I was dropping the inches. After a bit more searching around the internet I found this thing about inflammation, and how not giving your body time to recover from exercising is not a good thing. So I had to slow down. I was wondering why it took so long to lose inches. But I was overdoing it. I like pushing myself when I do exercises, and that means a lot of sweat and a lot of panting and puffing. And this little bit of information was probably the most important. My brother's son's friends are all into fitness and really into gyms, HITT Tabata style, and playing sports. One really fit dude is into competitive athletics and he is always sick. If there is a bug going round he'll get it. I thought he should be the healthiest of all of them but not so, he doesn't give his body time to recover from the constant grind of exercising. But he wants to win, so he has to do it or overdo it as he usually does. My brother's son is the same. I told him to slow down to give his body time to recover, but he keeps going and I must admit he is pretty fit, but he would be a lot healthier if he gave his body time to recover. This was the turning point for me but there was an accumulation of getting fitter before I arrived where I am now, and it did make a difference. Now I do a mixture of strength exercises and cardio, and I take days off to recover. If I have a spare bit of time or I have been sitting in front of the computer for too long, I'll do some karate katas just to break into sweat. Also there are some slow heavy breathing katas that are very good, where you are using concentration and strength as opposed to speed and power.

Doing Exercises In Other Cities

I'm now back on the road again, and that is not a good thing when you are trying to keep your weight under control. That means a lot of time on your butt, whether on airplanes or in airport stopovers. And the worst part is living of crap food and not drinking enough. And on top of that living in hotel rooms that are too small to do any exercises. I was in a dorm room with 4 other people, and there was no room to move let alone do any exercises. To top it off it was raining nearly everyday. I was in Hong Kong in the tropics in spring time. So I couldn't do any exercises in the park, like I used to do years ago when I was a lot younger and a lot fitter. Anyway I ended up walking up and down the stairs to the 16th floor twice a day. For a change I would go two stairs at a time for as many floors as I could. That made me feel real good, at least I was doing some exercise. I used to walk around the park in the rain with my umbrella, looking at the same spot where I used to do my exercises, hoping the rain would stop. But it didn't. Then I moved onto another city, still in the tropics and still raining. But this time I might go back to my gym and start up again. The only problem is I'm not sure how long I'll be staying here. There is one serious advantage with going to the gym here and that is most people doing workouts can speak English, as one foreigner found out the hard way. She was on the machine sweating it out and swearing her head off at the same time. Real colorful gutter language – you know "F this and F that and any other word she could throw in. Then one woman told her to stop swearing and everybody joined in and told her to shut up, they were very polite about it. Anyway the women never went back. You can assume anyone who can afford to go to the gym is very well educated, has a high paying job and speaks very good English. It is quite strange really, the English language in the west has deteriorated quite rapidly over the past 15 years or so, and in Asia and Russia they speak very good non gutter language. So in a foreign country be considerate what you say, when puffing and panting away on a machine.

Also here a few people are starting to run around the streets. The best time is early in the morning before the streets get clogged. I usually go to the park where I can run up and down the stairs and around the park. Just don't trip over any old ladies doing ti chi. Anyway you do a lot more walking here because you have too. And that includes climbing stairs on the walk bridges and walking up and down the stairs into the subway. And don't forget standing on the buses and trains. You are lucky if you can get a seat so I usually stand. So everyday you actually do a lot of exercises throughout the day. And the food is healthier to an extent, even though they have instant noodles nearly everywhere and MSG is in everything. I still do a workout in the afternoon, evening before I have a shower.

And here in the tropics you sweat all the time, so get used to it.

My afternoon workout consists mainly of simple cardio exercises interspaced with strength training. I do a lot of karate stuff like blocks and hits as hard and fast as I can, then I do the more mundane stuff like lunges and squats. After that it is on the floor for crunches, leg raises and pushups and whatever else I can think of. I usually end up with a plank. I get up a good sweat then have a shower. About 20 minutes each time. That is on top of all the walking and climbing stairs, so I keep very active.

Summary Time

When I started I had to get fit so I could exercise long enough to break out into sweat. And that took about a month. Then I had to settle into an exercise regime that I could do, and that I liked doing. That took another month, and I kept changing the exercises to find something that I could do and do for a reasonable length of time. I ended up doing HIIT (High Intensity Interval Training) with sprinting and jogging to recover, and fast skipping and jogging if it was raining. Then I'd do a round of exercise - lunges with a kick, squats with a punch (we do these at Karate) burpees, push-ups and finish off with a plank. Then I'd go for my cardio jog around the football field. And after all the exercises I felt pretty good when I was jogging, but I would only jog about six laps instead of ten. Other days I would go to self defense and fitness, and there we did a lot of ab work and heavy duty sweating as we practiced on the bags. There we did some very intense workouts like 20 push-ups, 20 leg raises, 20 situps, 20 squats then we would run to the other side of the gym and back and do it all again. We usually did three rounds before we started on the self defense.

There is a lot of stuff to wade through on the internet. But with the internet everything is quite handy, like just at your fingertips, and that can be a double edged sword with information overload. But it is very handy when you find out something new, you can dig deeper and decide whether to use the new information or not. And in most cases I changed my schedule to suit the new knowledge. Like I did when I found out about protein, I changed my exercise schedule to the afternoon to suit my eating habits or lack of eating habits. Then when I delved into recovery time, I changed my schedule again to accommodate the new information, and it all helped. So if you are not losing weight or inches and you are doing lots of exercises, check out the internet to find out why. You are in control of your own schedule, so have a look to see "Why" you are not doing so well.

Also just realize it takes time. You can't drop 10 years of indulgence in 10 days despite what you read on the internet. In my case, first I had to get fit so I could do the exercises long enough to have an effect. And after you are fitter, then you can start pushing yourself to lose weight. And that is when I started to feel good. So don't expect miracles, just keep plodding on.

I woke up one day and say my pot belly in the mirror and I thought 'Where did that come from.' I still think my main problem is the sleep connection. I still can't get over six hours of sleep a night. Even if I have an afternoon nap I just lay there and don't drop off. But with exercise and a decent diet I have managed to drop a few inches from around my waist. I am now just under a 36 inch waist which I haven't seen for over a year. I still eat biscuits and chocolate bars, but not as many as before. The only food I managed to stop eating was bread and butter.

The easiest way to lose weight is to go and live in the tropics in summer in a rather large city where you have to walk, climb stairs and stand on the subway and buses. And when it is 40 degrees C with humidity of over 90% you can't help but lost weight. Here the big plus is, you haven't got a car, and you have to carry a bag. And when you go shopping in the supermarket you have to carry your groceries home on the bus.

Things You Can Do

Here are a few things I kinder do naturally now to try and trim down.

- I try and park as far away as is reasonable to where I am going. In the supermarket and department store I try and park as far away from the entrance as possible. This way I have to at least walk somewhere. There are some inherent dangers in doing this. I was turning into a parking space just after I had entered the car park and the car behind me nearly crashed into me as they raced for the only parking space near the main doors.

- If I am doing a skype call or anything that involves talking and not sitting then I stand. I spend most of my time on my butt in front of the computer, so I try to stand at every opportunity I can. I actually looked at putting my computer on a higher desk to see if I could use it standing up. Not practical enough as typing is quite difficult. I might even look into these voice activated word programs to see if they would reduce sitting time. I used one years ago and it was not very good. Maybe the new generation will be more easier to correct.

- I love listening to educational and inspirational podcasts in my car. Now with mobile phones it is very easy to listen while you are driving. I never have the radio going while I am driving. My daughter will listen to her music with her earphones, and I will listen to my podcasts with my earphones on and everybody is happy. You can listen to audio books on diet and or how to do exercise. I don't recommend listening to meditation music, when you are driving that is not the right time.

- I don't own a TV, but if I had one I wouldn't be sitting in front of it after work, after sitting all day in front of a computer. I gave up the TV years ago and I don't miss it. Now with the internet I would say TV should be obsolete, but it is still hanging in there. If you are really into TV, put your exercise bike and other exercise machines in front of the TV instead of the sofa. Now you can do exercises while watching TV. As they say 'Kill two birds with one stone.'

- Now I have a slight problem with biscuits, chocolate and sweets, so I keep then out of sight. I have found that if I don't see them I don't want them. But then when my body is missing something, I will go through cupboards and the fridge looking for something to eat. So I keep hiding them in strange places. I vow never to buy biscuits again but as soon as I see them on special I buy heaps. The last time they were on special I brought about six packets. So that is something I have to work through.

- Another little tip I found on the internet is green tea has some type of fat reduction properties I've been drinking green tea for years. And maybe it helped keep me slim when I was living the life style, but after my life came unglued it didn't help.

Things I have not tried but sound pretty good.

- I drink green tea everyday but that is because I like it, I didn't realize it helped with weight loss. Anyway there are a few essential oils that are supposed to be quite effective against weight loss. And the one that stands out is peppermint oil as well as few others. With these essential oils you use the aroma so you need to be able to sniff them. If you are into this then try it out, and also if you are into new things you can give it a go too.

- If you are into color therapy you might try eating off blue plates, as blue is a color that suppresses appetite. I have never tried this but you can give it a go, everything helps.

One Thing To Be Very Careful Of.

I ended up with a hernia on my right side. Now be very careful because as you get older your body is starting to wear out and hernias can be caused by over exercising especially if you are doing weights. Now I don't know if my hernia was caused by over exercising or lifting something heavy or just the usual wear and tear as you get older.

The hernia was not very big so the doctors didn't worry about it. But then something happened after a year, and it suddenly tripled in size and people including my doctor and me started to worry. I kept exercising and that might have helped it to grow, so I stopped sit-ups and leg raises but I still do push-ups and the plank. Sit-ups and leg raises seemed to put more strain on the stomach muscles so I stopped doing them as they might have caused it to grow.

As you get older doctors used to worry about putting you under anesthetic to operate but now they don't seem to worry. The doctors want me to go in for an operation but I am very reluctant as I am not too keen on hospitals.

Be Careful About What You Read On The Internet

The internet is full of information but interspaced between the good stuff is a lot of rubbish. At one stage the internet related to getting fit was overrun with headings that basically said that running and or jogging was the worst exercise you could do. Now that is rubbish and after checking out a few of the sites it became obvious that they were all trying to sell some over priced fitness program that you could hardly do because you were not fit enough. And if you were jogging or running a little you would be a lot fitter, and you would be able to do their program. It has faded away now but it still pops up occasionally.

I don't know who started it or how it started but it took the fitness related internet by storm and because of the way Google runs its advertisements it was popping up every time you opened your computer. So as they say "Follow the money" and find out who is making the money then decide if you want to believe it or not. Most fitness people who promoted the idea that running was the worst exercise you could do somehow come to their senses and realized that any type of exercise is better than no exercise.

I did check out running to see if it was safe and it usually is but you have to be careful and not over do it. I thought my knees would pack up as I was running on concrete but running is actually good for your knees as long as your knees are not damaged when you start running. It might sound silly but movement helps your body from falling to bits as you get older and the movement in your knees when you are running helps to stop the damage. I used to use air shock shoes and other times I used anti shock inner soles and now I just use ordinary running shoes with no anti shock and so far my knees are good. You do not need to spend a lot of money on good shoes. I use cheap shoes now and my legs are good.

If You Are Not In Good Shape

Don't do silly things when you start. As has been said many time "You can't run before you can walk." So when you start a fitness program start by walking. I run around a small lake at lunch time in the hottest part of the day mainly because there are not many people at the lake at that time. Also another guy walks around very fast 4 times and he gets covered in sweat and he is getting fitter. Very soon he will start running. Another woman also walks around the lake at lunch time so start easy but you must put effort into the walking. After I've finished my run I'll walk with the guy and he walks fast so he is not there for a stroll. And that is what you must do. Put in the effort. We are all over 50 years old, so also you are never too old to start.

One More Thing

After I started losing weight I lost the fat and muscle but I still have folds of skin that I just can't seem to get rid of just hanging around my stomach. My boobs are just sagging there after the fat and muscle that used to fill them has been sweated away. When I am doing push-ups I look down my body and the folds of skin around my stomach and my boobs are just hanging there. Not a pretty sight and everything I have tried to get rid of it has done nothing. So when you get slim you might still have some unsightly folds hanging around your mid section.

What I Do Now

My maintenance program has changed a lot from the days of heavy exercise. When I run I try to run three to five kilometers, four to five times a week in summer and skipping in winter. I try to do HIIT twice a week with full on sprinting as hard as I can then slow jogging and walking until I can get my breath back and run again then I'm off again. I do this about two to three times a week depending on the weather. I still do push-ups and the plank but because of the hernia I do not do any crunches, sit-ups or leg raises but the hernia is still getting bigger so I might need to take a month off to get it repaired.

I now do Doctor Mercola's Nitric Oxide Dump which is a set of 4 exercises that are heart healthy. Now the time I spend on exercising is a lot less but other than the folds of skin I still manage to maintain a healthy weight to height ratio.

Articles From The Internet Mentioned In The Book

http://articles.mercola.com/sites/articles/archive/2010/04/29/green-tea-extract-effective.aspx

http://articles.mercola.com/sites/articles/archive/2015/04/23/green-tea-dementia.aspx

http://articles.mercola.com/sites/articles/archive/2014/09/03/too-much-protein.aspx

http://www.acaloriecounter.com/diet/calorie-deficit-to-lose-weight/

http://www.grassfedgirl.com/6-essential-oils-for-weight-loss/

http://realfoodswitch.com/raw-food-product-reviews/essential-oils-weight-loss-cravings/

http://www.colormatters.com/color-and-the-body/color-and-appetite-matters

http://www.aworkoutroutine.com/how-to-lose-fat-without-losing-muscle/

http://www.acaloriecounter.com/diet/pre-and-post-workout-meal/

http://www.acaloriecounter.com/diet/

http://fitness.mercola.com/sites/fitness/archive/2016/01/15/stand-up-sit-less-move-more.aspx?

http://fitness.mercola.com/sites/fitness/archive/2016/02/12/extreme-exercise-affects-heart.aspx?

http://www.thealternativedaily.com/staying-up-late-can-make-you-fat/?

http://www.ncbi.nlm.nih.gov/pmc/articles/PMC535701/

https://fitness.mercola.com/sites/fitness/archive/2018/08/10/why-you-need-to-try-the-nitric-oxide-dump-workout.aspx

Exercise Videos

https://www.youtube.com/watch?v=Sg3CTnoFXDA

https://www.youtube.com/watch?v=WLx5q7M741k

https://www.youtube.com/watch?v=2k9fUP7_MWI

If You Like My Book

Please write a review on Amazon showing your appreciation

How to Write a Review on Amazon

- Go to https://www.amazon.com/dp/B01FB3FC3K

- Scroll down to Customer Reviews

- Click on "Write a customer review" and do your thing. As long or as short as you like.

Amazon will then check it and after a while it will be live on Amazon.Now you can give the book a grade, 5 Gold Stars would be lovely.

Thank you

Peter LeGrove

Other Books By Peter LeGrove

Teach and Travel in China

This little book is all about going to China and getting a job teaching English. Even though it is Guangzhou specific it still covers little things that could happen in China. A good read if you are heading out into the world to travel.

Live And Teach In Vietnam

If you are looking for country where you can "Live Cheap In An UnCheap World" then Vietnam should be on your radar. This little book tells you about life as it is on the streets of Vietnam, and how to get a job, place to stay and what ever else you need.

How To Teach Young Learners ESL

This book is an accumulation of my seven years of classroom teaching, face to face with kids from kindergarten to the end of primary school. This is what worked for me, and it has been distilled from lots of stuff that didn't work. So you end up with the crème de la crème. Teaching kids is the way to go, if you are into teaching and traveling.

Reading Student Struggling Student

If you are not into leaving your child in front of the computer to learn to read, then this book is for you. This is a hands on approach to teaching your child to read, using a method that has been teaching children to read for over a hundred years. And it is still applicable in this internet age.

Prepare Now To Survive Mother Nature's Wrath Or Mankind's Madness

At present in the world, there is a group of people who think the world is heading for a major collapse. And on the other side, there has been an increase in what Mother Nature can do to the planet. This book is about common sense preparing for what could happen without going overboard.

How To Add Qualifications To Your CV Using FREE Courses

To add more color to your CV, and to help give you the edge in the job market. Fill up the spaces with certificates from free courses run by world renowned universities. There is a whole new world of free education out there in cyberspace, you just have to plug into and this little book shows you where it all is.

How To Make An Online CV Using Free Software

With the internet taking over our lives it is only a matter of time before you apply for an online job using an Online CV. In this little book you will learn how to put together a professional Online CV using only FREE software freely available over the internet. Also what you learn can be adapted to online presentations as well.

Prepare Your Children For The Future NOW

The world with the internet is changing so fast now it is very difficult to keep up. So to keep your children ahead of the curve you need to start them early on the internet. This way when they are ready to head out into the New World of cyberspace they are already over half way there.

Live Cheap In An UnCheap World

For some reason the world we live in is getting more and more expensive, so now it is time to change. To make your money last longer, you either have to tighten your belt, make more money or do things differently. Now this little books shows you ways to do all three so you can end up with more money at the end of the week.

Thank you and all the best on your journey into getting trim and more healthy. Jut remember it takes time and effort and I don't think there is any way to short cut the process.

Peter Legrove

reader are responsibility for your actions and safety while trying to lose some belly fat.

www.ingramcontent.com/pod-product-compliance
Lightning Source LLC
Chambersburg PA
CBHW032102280526
45784CB00013B/2994